Reiki Manual

Level Three

Rajesh Nanoo

For orders and enquires, contact
www.rajeshnanoo.com
mrknowable@gmail.com

Reverence be,
O Prana,
To thee coming,
Reverence to thee going;
Reverence to thee standing &
Reverence, too,
To thee sitting!

Atharva Veda

Dr. Rajesh Nanoo MD(AM) had a spiritual inclination from my early days towards occult sciences and music. At first he nurtured his skills in Multimedia and started creating logos, posters and storyboard for various clients. Shortly his attention shifted to the potentials of Reiki and embraced this astonishing healing power. With enthusiasm, he pursued this magnificent profession along with Yoga Therapy and learned other holistic techniques which enabled him to hasten the healing process.

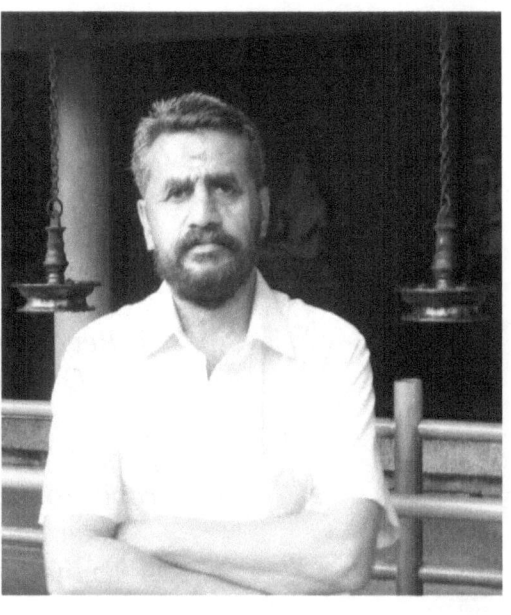

The research done on various philosophies enabled him to come up with training modules on enhancing life skills. He was involved in training people on the secret of working smartly, giving energy healing and teaching relaxation techniques to withstand the stress of the modern society.

Holistic training/healing methodology is a self-help tool to pull us out from difficulties; it has an integral part to play in character making. Rajesh Nanoo have comprehended this truth and crave to extend this awareness for the needy ones for cure and also to renovate their character, thereby let the world recognize the new era of healing/training that has begun by transcending a man completely.

CONTENTS

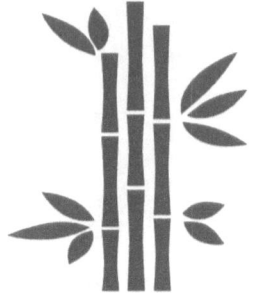

1

Ethics Of The Master

A Reiki master has to fulfill two obligations. First obligation is towards the lineage so he should indulge on those things that corrupt it. Second obligation is to pass on the techniques to the competent student so that this healing methodology will not be lost again. Only limited ethics are outlined for a Reiki master because he has reached in a higher state, which declares, "I am Reiki. It is not an ego-building statement. It is so because his intellect and Reiki's intellect came into a union, only then he is qualified for the coveted Reiki Master Level. Hence it will be blasphemy to teach him lot of ethics. Still there is some etiquette to follow:

1. Master should act as a synthesis of Reiki teachings, practical healing and esoteric knowledge.
2. Never remain reluctant in giving initiation to a qualified student.
3. Never refrain from initiation due to unnecessary or silly reasons particularly occurred due to his ego with the student.
4. Never exchange Reiki as a shortcut to be rich. Reiki has higher values, which cannot be traded by money. Thus the benefits and its value cannot be measured in the weigh of money. Hence, never be greedy with money.
5. Never make distinction between students by money or assets they have. Treat every one equally.
6. Reiki master should respect each student's right to choose their own healing path and their masters.
7. Never feel jealousy and become reluctant to admire the great Reiki masters living around the globe.

8. Never feel jealousy towards his students incase if they surpass him in mastery of practice and application of Healing.

9. Never think that the student has an obligation to you in their whole life. We should remain unattached, because the choice is left to the student whether he admire you or not. The outcome (good or bad) of the student's behavior will solemnly affect the student, thus no need to heed on such trivial matters.

10. When a master thinks that, by giving initiation he will loose his priority over the patients or students is an irrational thinking and against the ethics of the Reiki. Reiki technique was lost in olden times because of such selfish thinking. So it is a prime obligation to Prana and Usui to transfer our knowledge for the benefit of others. Keep in mind that we obtained Reiki because Usui transferred to other competent masters; if Usui were reluctant to transfer then this technique would have lost again. Similarly the masters in our lineage too have passed this methodology. Hence it is our responsibility to transfer this to others.

11. Never initiate a student if he does not posses faith in it. It is good to give Reiki session to those who do not have any faith, after two or three sessions they will understand what Reiki is, but never teach some one who neither have faith or respect Reiki.

12. Give initiation (first and second) only to sincere, honest, simple and dedicated persons

13. Students should not be stubborn; they should have a reasonable understanding and intellect so they can comprehend the subtle philosophies. I am not saying that student should be an extraordinary person but he should be bright enough to understand the procedures of symbols, sessions.

14. Give master degree only to those person who are sincere, honest, and posses enough healing experience. This is very important because only such a student have the capacity to transfer energy to other. He should also comprehend

the procedures and intricacies of attunements and energy enhancement.

15. Reiki master should mainly hand over the information given by Mikao Usui through his lineages. There is no harm in teaching philosophies that are aligning towards Reiki methodology. The only criteria are, in such cases the other materials should be introduced clearly as an additional from traditional ambit of Reiki teachings.

16. Always keep the traditional methods intact while adding new methods in initiation. Other methodologies should only be add on.

17. Follow the traditional yardstick of intervals while first, second and master level initiations.

18. He should give all the necessary information about Reiki methodology and also give symbols in its exact form to the students. Do not hide any information from them so as to sustain your dominance.

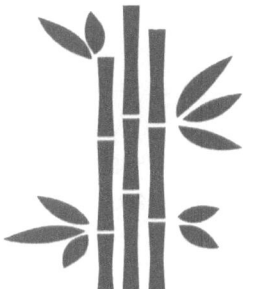

2

Food Combination

Proper combination of food is very much important to keep vital energies intact and also for keeping himself away from diseases. A Reiki master should always be vigilant about his food habits and also that of the patients. Upanishad says Annam Bramheti means - Food is a Creator. This means that we living beings are creation of food which clearly indicates that we are what we Eat.

Our diet is an essential factor for the formation of our body. It is clearly mentioned in classic Ayurvedic text Charak samhita that consuming improper diet in improper way is the main cause of disease.

According to Charak samhita: "An appropriate and suitable diet in a disease is equivalent to hundred drugs and any quantity of drug hardly compares to good results in disease without following proper dietetic regimen". In as far as diet is concerned, Ayurveda has recommended the following principles for living full span of life with perfect health.

The intake of diet and what you should take and should not depends upon a number of factors, among which, surprisingly includes the desha or territory), kala or season, and time of the day etc. You should consume foods belonging to all six rasas or tastes rather than just a few of them so as to avoid nutritional deficiency disorders. Various tastes provide you different nutrients.

Ayurveda & Six Tastes (Shad Rasas)

In Ayurvedic method, food is classified by the effect it has on our body. There are six primary tastes in Ayurvedic cuisine, each representing different types of foods that play individual roles in balancing your dosha. Sweet tastes have a strengthening effect, sour tastes stimulate the digestive system, salty tastes maintain your water and electrolyte balance, pungent tastes improve digestion and absorption of nutrients, astringent tastes also help with absorption and bitter taste stimulates all other tastes. Understanding them and how they relate to our individual constitution can help us make better choices to promote and maintain health.

According to Ayurveda, we are born with a unique constitution, which is an individual combination of the three Doshas, or principles that govern the function of our bodies on the physical, mental and emotional levels. These three energies are Vata, Pitta & Kapha. Disease is caused by an imbalance of any of the doshas and by the presence of ama, or toxic food byproducts (foods which are not digested) According to Ayurveda, the best preventive medicine and support of the natural healing process is a diet & lifestyle specific to the constitutional needs of the individual.

Time of consuming food:

A person should take meal only when he feels hungry. Lunch should be taken early between 12 noon to 1afternoon; a time that coincides with the peak pitta period. Pitta is responsible for the digestion. Lunch should be the largest meal of the day. The supper should be lesser and lighter than lunch. .

Quantity of food:

Generally half of the capacity of stomach should be filled with solids, one-fourth with liquids and rest kept empty for the free movements of body humors. That means you should actually get up when you feel you should eat a little, just a little more! Sequence of consuming food is given below.

Madhur or sweet rasa food like fruits are advisable for intake in the beginning of meal, food with amla and lavana (sour and salty) rasa in the middle and katu, tikta, kashay (bitter, astringent and pungent) foods should be taken at the end of the meal.

Method of consuming food:

1) Wash the face, hands and feet before meal. Dine in an isolated neat and clean place in pleasant environment. Squat/sit rather than stand while you eat.

2) Food should be taken after complete digestion of previous one.

3) Hard items should be consumed in the beginning followed by soft and liquids subsequently.

4) Few sips of water are advised now and then while taking meal.

5) Heavy substances are contraindicated after meals and should be avoided.

6) Consumption of excessively hot food leads to weakness. Cold and dry food leads to delay in digestion. Intake of food prepared by giving extra heat leads to glani; hence consumption of such food should be avoided.

Tips for eating:

There is a beautiful passage in the Sanskrit literature describing all types of foods and their actions. Among the digestive aids referred there are the following:

1. Water, which imparts a liquid quality and helps in digestion and absorption of food.
2. Salt also aids digestion, and helps to retain water.
3. Alkalies help digestion and regulate gastric fire (HCL).
4. Ghee stimulates agni and improves digestion.
5. Milk invigorates.
6. Meat gives energy. Also in this literature are descriptions on influence of foods on the tri-dosha:

1. Pitta is increased by foods, which are sour and pungent.
2. Kapha is aggravated by milk products.
3. Vata is over-stimulated by beans, dry fruits, astringent and bitter substances.

The daily diet should contain:

- 40 & 50% well-cooked basmati rice, barley, corn or wheat depending upon one is constitution.
- 15 - 30% well cooked legumes.
- 2 - 5% vegetable soups.
- 1/2-teaspoon pickles

In order to stimulate appetite one can chew and eat 1/2-teaspoon fresh grated ginger with a pinch of rock salt before each meal.

Ayurveda insists that iced water should not be drunk during or after a meal as it slows agni and digestion. Small sips of warm water taken during the meal serves to aid digestion. While eating one should properly masticate the food in order to soften it and ensure that it is thoroughly mixed with saliva. If desired, one can finish a meal by drinking a cup of lassi (or takram). This can be made by blending four teaspoons of yogurt with two pinches of ginger and cumin powder in one cup of water.

When eating, only one third of the capacity of the stomach should be filled with food, one-third with liquid and one third should be left empty. This will aid in proper digestion and also promotes mental clarity.

Incompatible Food Combinations

Milk Is Incompatible With:
Acidic foods, Salty foods, fish, Meat, Radish, Garlic,Drumstick, Honey,mango,orange,banana,jackfruit,coconut,pomegranate, sour foods. gooseberry, beans, white pumpkin, urd gram, mushroom, gingelly, curd, yoga hurt, oil, sprouted cereals, dried fruits, wine, Melons, Bread containing yeast, Cherries.

Melons Are Incompatible With:
Grains, Starch, Fried foods, Cheese

Starches Are Incompatible With:
Eggs, Tea, Milk, Bananas, Dates, Persimmons

Honey Is Incompatible With:
- Ghee (in equal proportions)
- Hot water and hot foods
- Oily foods
- Honey followed by hot water and radish is also forbidden

Radishes Are Incompatible With:
Milk, Bananas, Raisins, Nightshades,

(Potato, Tomato, Eggplant, Chilies) Are Incompatible With:
Yogurt, Milk, Melon, Cucumber

Yogurt/Curd Is Incompatible With:
Milk, Sour Fruits, Melons, Hot drinks, Meat, Fish, Mangos, Starch, Cheese

Eggs Are Incompatible With:
Milk, Meat, Yogurt, Melons, Cheese, Fish, Bananas

Mangoes Are Incompatible With:
Yogurt, Cheese, Cucumbers
Corn Is Incompatible With:
Dates, Raisins, Bananas

Lemon Is Incompatible With:
Yogurt, Milk, Cucumbers, Tomatoes

Meat and fish are incompatible and also incompatible with:
Honey, Gingelly oil, jaggery, milk, dal, radish, sprouted cereals,
fatty foods.

Other Wrong Food Combinations

- The food that has a Sour taste should not be mixed with the food that has salt, chilly hot, bitter, brackish taste
- The foods that have a sweet taste should not be mixed with salt, chilly hot, bitter and brackish taste
- Salty foods should not be mixed with chilly hot, bitter, brackish taste
- Fatty food along with rainy water
- Meat, milk, honey should not be mixed with mustard oil
- Sugar and fish is incompatible
- Raw meat with wine is incompatible
- Banana and urdgram is incompatible
- Dates and banana is incompatible
- Bitter and brackish is incompatible
- Sugar jaggery and radish is incompatible
- Curd and banana is incompatible

General rules about food consumption:

1. Walk a while after meal to help digestion
2. No traveling, exercise or sexual intercourse within one hour after meal.

3. Avoid meals when thirsty and water while hungry.
4. Avoid meals after exertion.
5. Avoid meals when you are having no appetite.
6. Don't suppress the appetite as it leads to body pain, anorexia, lassitude, vertigo and general debility.
7. Don't suppress the thirst as it leads to general debility, giddiness and heart diseases.
8. Consumption of the fresh, acceptable, easily available and compatible food with various nutrients is a key to lead a healthy life.

Antidotes for Incompatible Food Combination

Proper combination of food substances, keeping in view the 5 factors given in the previous article, can enhance the process of digestion and aid in nutrition of body. If the negative effects of food items are known, they can be made wholesome by combining them with appropriate counteracting food items or "antidotes" as given below:

1. Cheese increases congestion and mucous. It aggravates pitta and kapha. To counteract this, you can add black pepper.
2. Eggs in cooked form increase pitta, and in raw form, increase kapha. Turmeric and onions are the antidotes.
3. Ice cream increases mucous and causes congestion. If taking ice cream is inevitable, then top it with clove and cardamom.
4. Curd increases mucous and causes congestion. Cumin and ginger will take care of the ill effects of curd.
5. Fish increases pitta. Coconut, lime and lemon are the remedial measures to counteract the bad effects of fish.
6. Meat is heavy to digest. Cloves or pepper powder makes the digestion easier.

7. Alcohol has both stimulating and depressing effects. Chewing a pinch of cumin seeds or 1-2 cardamom seeds may minimize these undesirable effects.

8. The bad effects of tea can be lessened with ginger. In the same way, ill effects of coffee can be kept at bay with nutmeg powder.

9. It is a known fact that sweets increase congestion. Addition of dry ginger powder (Sonthi/soonth) to the sweetmeats will decrease the congestion.

10. Tobacco aggravates pitta and stimulates vaata. Brahmi, calamus root (vasa/vacha) are used as antidotes to tobacco.

11. Rice and wheat increase kapha and fat. Clove and ginger are used to enhance the beneficial effects of these cereals.

12. Legumes produce gas and distention. Garlic, cloves, black pepper, ginger, rock salt or chili powder are the antidotes.

13. Cabbage produces gas due to its sulphur content. Cook in sunflower oil adding turmeric and mustard seeds.

14. Garlic increases pitta. Grated coconut and lemon counteract this effect.

15. Green salad produces gas. Cooking reduces the gas formation but, at the same time, its therapeutic benefits may also be lost. If you want to have salad in raw form, add a little quantity of lemon juice to it.

16. Onion also produces gas. To prevent this either you should take it in cooked form or you should add salt, lemon, and curd and mustard seed powder to it.

17. Potato, due to its high carbohydrate content, produces gas. This can be reduced with ghee and pepper.

18. Tomato increases kapha. Lime and cumin are the antidotes to it.

19. The ill effects like increase in kapha of banana can be counteracted with cardamom.
20. Mango some times produces diarrhea. Adding ghee with cardamom is the remedy.
21. Melon causes water retention. Grated coconut with coriander is the solution to this.
22. Most people who consume nuts and peanuts, experience gas and burning sensation in the stomach. As a remedial measure, either you should soak them overnight or cook them with sesame oil, ginger, roasted cumin powder and pepper.

Food combination is robbing the joy of eating these days. Thus enjoy varieties of roods by planning your food menu.

* Note: This article is taken from various Ayurveda website and combine together for better understanding and bringing various topic under one umbrella.

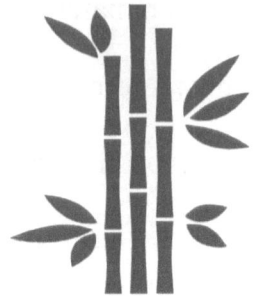

3

Master Symbols

There are two symbols in the master degree and there is another three non traditional master symbols. The two master symbols are given below.

1. Master symbol (DKM).

Translation: may the great light shine

According to our view light is the source of knowledge. All the knowledge we have grasped is obtained via flashes, which is a form of light. The light destroys ignorance and darkness. Hence we can interpret DKM as - let the knowledge blossoms (in the head). The symbol is empowered with the vibration of great lights

*History of the symbol**

The complete phrase 'DKM' appears as part of a sacred 'nine-syllable' mantra dating from before the 8thC: "Shiken Haramitsu Daikomyo" which conceptually translates as: "The Wisdom of the Four Hearts* leads us to Enlightenment. The Merciful Heart expresses love for everything, the Sincere Heart follows, what is right, the Attuned Heart follows the natural order of things, and the Dedicated Heart holds to the chosen pursuit.

It also occurs in the name: "DKM-O" - 'Great Shining Bright King'. DKM- O is one of the daison myo-o (great and venerable kings of magic knowledge) - compassionate yet wrathful deities who protect humans against evil influences, and who possess the knowledge and force contained in mantras.

In one respect, just as the siddham character Kiriku is regarded as itself possessing the divine grace of the Buddha it represents, so too in an esoteric sense, the three-kanji phrase 'DKM' may be seen to directly represent the mystical experience of Komyo [the 'Bright Light' or 'Enlightened Nature': the Radiance of a given Deity], and as such, may be employed by one who has achieved that 'enlightenment,' as a means of passing on (- to a lesser degree -) the effects of that experience to others.

Note – Taken from various Internet sources

2. TIBETAN MASTER SYMBOL(TM)

Translation: awakening of the Prana.

I assume that the symbol is originated from the Tibetan masters. This symbol is also powerful as DKM. Usui/ Tibetan folks call the "non-traditional DKM" or the "Tibetan DKM is actually the Tibetan Medicine Buddha Symbol called "Dumo". It has a much different meaning the master symbol DKM of Usui system. Although some have claimed that TM is the "goddess spiral" its tradition is drawn from Tibetan Medicine Buddha practices and not from Wiccan religion based faiths. While the form of the symbol really matters little, the intent of Usui system was based on the understanding of DKM, not on the Tibetan DKM that others added into the system. This symbol is given to the master on Reiki Teacher Level (The Fourth)

(Note: Our TM has got a variation from this Dumo. Only in the top most part of the TM has the shape of Demo. Hence we cannot actually say that this is the Dumo symbol.

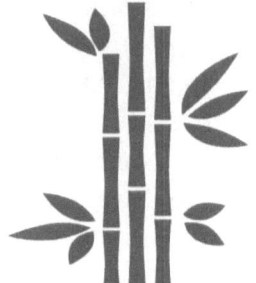

4

Nontraditional Symbols

TM is a mixture of CKR and Dumo.)

The three non traditional symbols Dumo, Raku and Fire dragon; is the mixture of TM, some of the masters draw them separately. The effectiveness is the same of TM.

1. Anthakarana -Ancient Symbol of Healing

The symbol did not exist in Usui Reiki, it may have a "Tibetan" origin and is most ancient. The symbol has a resemblance of Swastika, which is the most universal among symbols. Saints from yore used swastika for obtaining peace. Anthakarana symbol is drawn in the hands while sweeping and removes negative energies of patients or students in initiations. Some person use the symbol to cleanse crystals from negative energy obtained through crystal healing. The symbol is also

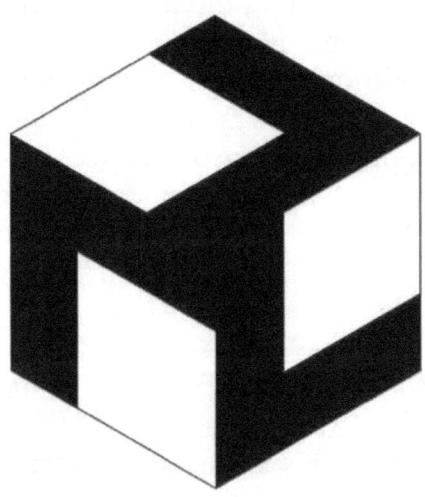

good for visualization.

Anthakarana Visualization*

The visualization practice included here is attributed to Tibetan practices. It is said that the monks would use a room lit with seven candles. An earthen vessel would be in the room. Its shape was oval. It contained water. The oval shaped vessel represented the "cosmic egg" of the universe. There was a stool that the monk would sit upon, which contained the Anthakarana symbol made out of silver metal. Purportedly the monks would sit on the stool and meditate on the Reiki symbols, which were on a copper mirror on the other side of the room, which would merge the heavenly Reiki energies, and the Anthakarana would focus the earth energy blending them in the chakras.

*Note – Taken from Internet sources

2. Raku (Rah Koo)

This symbol is also not from Usui system; hence it is an addition to traditional Reiki teachings. The Buddhist and Shinto priests use this symbol, as a gesture to end rituals hence it was probably adapted from it. It has a shape of lightning. I believe that the Symbol inside TM is this symbol, so no needs to use Raku separately. It is commonly used at the start of attunements.

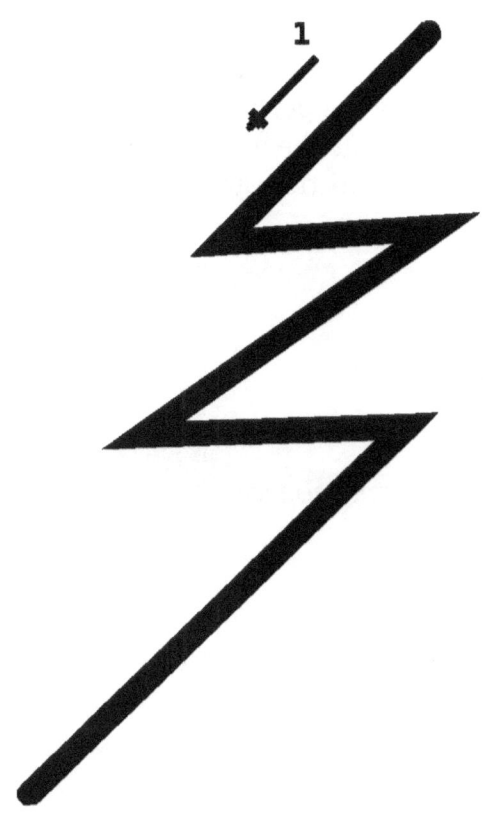

3. Fire Dragon or Fire Serpent

      This symbol is also not from Usui system; hence it is an addition to traditional Reiki teachings. When the TM is drawn in the hand it has this shape of fire serpent, so no need to draw Fire Dragon symbol separately.

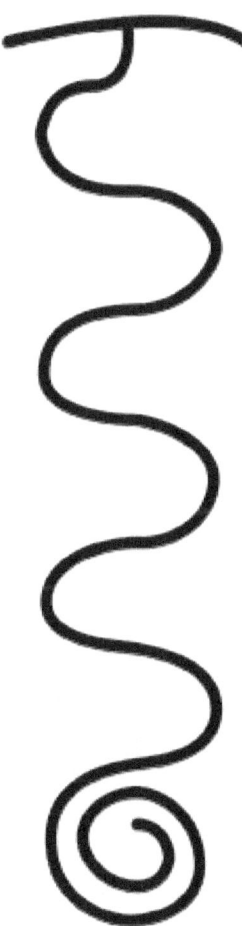

4. Dumo

The symbol, DUMO, is pronounced as "do moe". It represents the swirling fiery heat of the Kundalini. It is thought to be the igniter of the Sacred Flame or Kundalini fire.

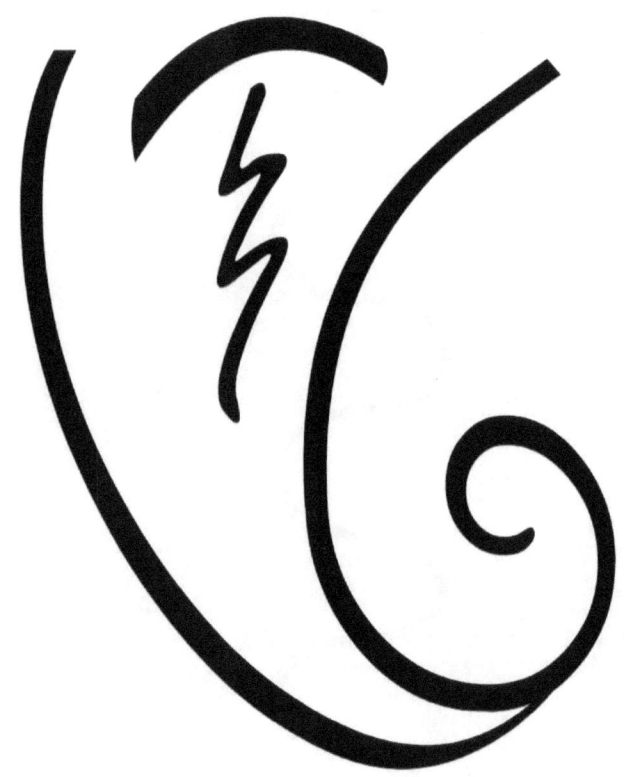

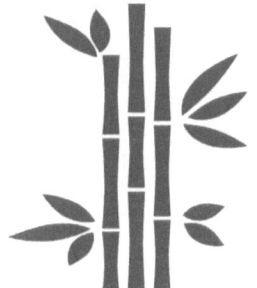

5

Reiki Session

Clear the negative energy in the room by drawing a huge CKR in the room and bed either by hand or by stick (which used to smudge). Then protect your self by smudging the aura by DKM. Then smudge the aura of the patient by DKM in the front and CKR in the back.

Ask him to lie comfortably in the bed. Draw Anthakarana symbol in your hand and sweep the negative energy of the patient. After that draw Raku symbol in your hand and move towards the space in between legs and give a little energy in the aura. The negative energy is absorbing through hands and going deep to the earth.

Then move to the head area, draw DKM in your hand and place one hand above (to the sky) as receiving energy from there and place the other hand into the patient's head and give energy. Let the negative energy be replaced with the positive energy. Then go and wash your hands if needed.

Draw DKM and chant the name. Visualize all the 4 symbols in front of you and it is entering into your heart one by one. Now you are personified with heavenly vital energy. Place your hands on the eyes (first position) and begin the treatment. Use CKR, SHK, HSZSN on all parts that is needed.

After the treatment session finished, first do stoke. After that feel in mind that energy is balanced or you can balance with the hands. Then seal the energy with CKR. Draw the DKM in the patient's aura and give little energy. Now the session is closed.

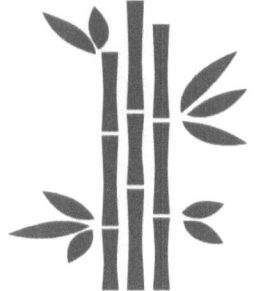

6

Psychic Surgery

This technique is not that of Usui Reiki system. It is also an addition to Reiki healing. Psychic surgery is a phrase with many meanings. For some people it refers as clearing negative energy out of the energy field from the body. For some others it means the removal of thought forms. For some others it refers to processes such as the removal of memory imprints or soul retrieval. In areas such as the Philippines psychic surgery means the literal physical removal of cysts or tumors from inside the body using hands sans cutting instruments.

We can use this technique on a regular Reiki session or do it independently. All diseases are mainly due to the mental blocks. In some cases we need to remove these blocks using psychic surgery rather than a Reiki session. This will result in faster healing, which is much more than normal healing. Do this only when you have full confidence and perform it meticulously. The entire process is very much delicate and requires high skills so if there is no confidence in doing it then the results wont be positive.

Thought forms can either be positive or negative. Negative thought forms brings illnesses of different types. Since the origin of thoughts is mind, it is the mind to be healed. It is healed by the same mind, which had the negative thoughts before because the power to over come also comes from the inner mind. The only difference is this power was slept before what is needed to overcome this.

Thought forms of both natures arouse from the conscious as well as the unconscious mind. In awaken state the unconscious mind is mostly in the sleeping mode. In the sleep state (of nights) the unconscious mind is awakened, this is known to us in the form of dreams. The power of the unconscious mind is infinite.

When the unconscious mind is awakened through conscious suggestions miraculous results happen. Positive thoughts can be bought in by various ways this will clear out the negative thoughts. Suggestion (by oneself or others) is a way to bring up the positive thought forms. A powerful suggestion evokes a special power that enables the person to overcome negative thoughts, which at one time lead to depression or psychic disorders. A psychic surgery combined with Reiki energy bestows amazing positive results.

The whole procedure is very simple because a patient will have a weaker mind while the healer have stronger mind. During the treatment the healer gains mastery over the patient's mind. Through this powerful mind the healer destroys the problem of the patient. All issues or thoughts do have forms. It may have a shape, weight or color, etc. Thus the problem is matched with that form or there is strong link between the both. The healer chooses an imaginary weapon to destroy these forms and freed the patient from his problems.

The Method to do

First ask the patient the issue they want to heal. Note that, it is not necessary for them to tell you what exactly the issue is. So tell them to imagine the issue themselves than telling to the healer. This can be very helpful for many patients because some issues are so sensitive that they do not want anyone to know about them.

Once the issue is put into thought, ask them in which part of the body they feels the problem is, has it got a shape, if so how is it looking like. Once they reply fathom into it. If they reply that there is no shape then ask them about its color if there is any. These quires are raised to know the nature of the problem. If there is no particular answer for both questions then ask for the weight or sound into which the problem is attached. Healer will definitely get an answer to one of those questions. Ask them are they interested to heal it and if the answer is yes then tell them that you're going to heal them with powerful Reiki rays.

Draw the master symbols in the hand and chant their names as in a regular treatment. Draw CKR on the front of our body for protection and draw on each chakra for better result. Use your inner mind any methods to destroy the problem with an imaginary weapon like sword, knife, hammer, flame etc. The healer should fathom deeply about the problem deeply and search a suitable instrument to destroy it. I normally use a trident. Once the instrument is selected then throw it (trident) to the form (that is mentioned by the patient). This weapon will destroy and take away the form from their body.

In this destructive process make harder sounds like "haa, hoo, hum. Etc. so that the patient too feels the form is getting destroyed. Tell them the form is getting burned or destroyed moment by moment and finally it is fully gone. After that, ask the patient whether he is still seeing that form he complained is solved or not?

The problem, which had shape, color, texture, weight, sound etc. is still there or not. If they say it is all gone ask them is there anything else remain that is to be sort out. If there is any then remove that too in similar fashion. After Psychic surgery some may feel positive forms in the place of negative forms. Some feel a vacuum. In both cases the surgery is success. After the psychic surgery full body treatment is good.

Suppose if they say the problem is not gone then repeat the process till it gets destroyed. In some cases the form may not change but the place in which the problem lied may vary. You have to remove the negative substance irrespective of its position. There can be invisible codes between the patient and the healer; this is chopped away by cutting it. This destruction will be good if it is like that of karate movements, using similar positive sounds.

The Healer can also imagine that he is stretching his fingers (of both hands) approximately 12 to 18 inches. With these extended fingers take out the problematic form from the patient's body and send it to the sky. Repeat this procedure till the patent sure that he is cured. After the surgery imagine that the fingers are restored back to its normal position.

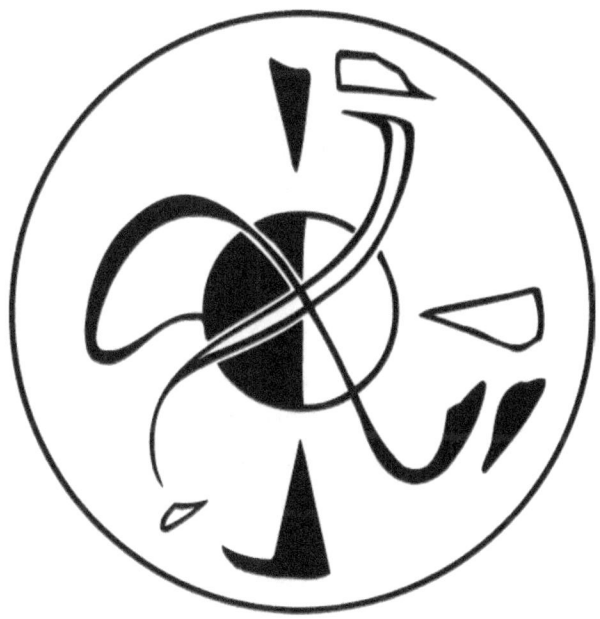

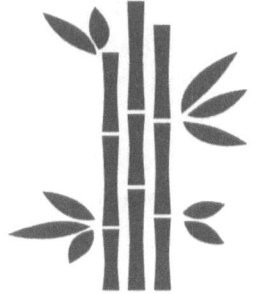

7

Visualizations

Energy Visualization

It is an old technique as found within the esoteric traditions of Tibetan & Japanese Buddhism. Assume a posture that's comfortable. Do Pranayama. Concentrate on mind and allow thoughts and feelings arise and pass away, without evaluation.

Relax your body and open your heart. The transparent, golden light-energy in the bubbles grows sharper and clearer now. Inside the bubbles, a radiant DKM symbol glows, and a beam of golden light enters your forehead. Feel the inner vibration of the DKM symbol and whole body is filled with it. It purifies all the four levels and dissolving all disturbing impressions in brain, nerves and senses. All causes and karmic imprints of harmful actions diminish and you feel your entire body relax.

Repeat the same procedure with CKR, SHK and HSZSN and feel their inner vibrations. Remain there as long as you wish. All effort, visualization and thought dissolve. Concentrate in a formless state of mind, without any frame of reference, without any conceptual elaboration, simply allowing your mind to rest in that state of delight with the amalgamation of Reiki energy. Now the mind is full of sublime level of energy.

Master degree symbol visualization

Sit calmly with head upright, and eyes closed. Chant OM three times. You can use any other Mantras instead of OM as per your religious upbringing. After that, watch your breath, inhaling and exhaling. Imagine that through every breath you are tuning with this source. That divine energy is inhaled to stomach and exhaled from there. Draw CKR in front of your body (a few inches away from face) Draw SHK in your right side and HSZSN on back Raku on left side. Draw Dumo above your head and Anthakarana below the foot. Imagine white rays of energy are coming from all parts and negative energy is oozing out through legs.

After that draw DKM in your heart. It is glazing in golden light rays. The energy emits from is like the rays of sun. This fills the heart with positive energy and later on spreading to other parts of the body. Now inside and outside the body is filled with positive energy or you are in middle of world, which is surrounded by positive energy. Remain like that till you feel enough. Then do Pranayama a few times and chant OM three times or the Mantra chanted before the meditation. Slowly open your eyes.

There is one more way to do Symbol meditation, which I normally teach in my class and also lots of ancient practices in Tibetan and Yogic system for Reiki Second level. Those techniques are not mentioned in the manual because it should be taught and monitored by a competent master. Get in touch with me to know more about it.

Reiki Moving Meditation

Stand straight with legs apart and hands folded in Gassho position. Stretch your hands a few inches away from your body but still in Gassho. After that slowly draw DKM with both hands with Gassho position. Separate the hands, move upwards and hold both hand above your head (palm facing upward) and say:

"I am receiving the vital energy form the cosmos". Bring down both hands in a rotating fashion and hold the palm downwards and say "I accept the energy and established it in my body as well as in the earth. Draw all three Reiki symbols and repeat the procedure. After that remain silent for a minute and then back to normal.

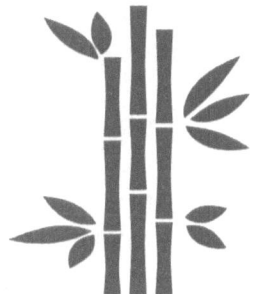

8

Additional Materials

Lectures from Swami Vivekananda

Note: These are complete lectures extracted form complete works of Swami Vivekananda. Read Raja yoga translated by Swamiji for further details. If you go through this thoroughly then there will never be even a slight doubt regarding the efficiency of healing by Prana.

Prana

The theory of creation is that matter is subject to five conditions: ether, luminous ether, gaseous, liquid, and solid. They are all evoked out of one primal element, which is very finest ether. The name of the energy in the universe is Prana, which is the force residing in these elements. Mind is the great instrument for using the Prana. Mind is material. Behind the mind is Atman which takes hold of the Prana. Prana is the driving power of the world, and can be seen in every manifestation of life.

The body is mortal and the mind is mortal; both, being compounds, must die. Behind all is the Atman which never dies. The Atman is pure intelligence controlling and directing Prana. But the intelligence we see around us is always imperfect. When intelligence is perfect, we get the Incarnation—the Christ. Intelligence is always trying to manifest itself, and in order to do this it is creating minds and bodies of different degrees of development. In reality, and at the back of all things, every being is equal. Mind is very fine matter; it is the instrument for manifesting Prana. Force requires matter for manifestation.

The next point is how to use this Prana. We all use it how sadly we waste it! The first doctrine in the preparatory stage is that all knowledge the outcome of experience. Whatever is beyond the five senses must also be experienced in order to become true to us. Our mind is acting on three planes: the subconscious, conscious and super conscious.. Of men, the Yogi alone is super conscious. The whole theory of Yoga is to go beyond the mind. These three planes can be understood.

These three planes can be understood by considering the vibrations of light or sound. There are certain vibrations of light too slow to become visible; then as they get faster, we see them as light; and then they get too fast for us to see them at all. The same with sound. How to transcend the senses without disturbing the health is what we want to learn. The Western mind has fumbled into acquiring some of the psychic gifts which .in them are abnormal and are frequently the sign of disease. The Hindu has studied and made perfect this subject of science, which all may now study without fear or danger.

Mental healing is a fine proof of the super conscious state; for the thought which heals is a sort of vibration in the Prana, and it does not go as a thought but as something higher for which we have no name. Each thought has three states. First, the rising or beginning, of which we are unconscious; second, when the thought rises to the surface; and third, when it goes from us, thought, is like a bubble rising to the surface. When thought is joined to will, we call it power. That which strikes the sick person whom you are trying to help is not thought, but power. The self-man running through it all is called in Sanskrit Sutratma, the "Thread-self".

The last and highest manifestation of Prana is love. The Moment you have succeeded in manufacturing love out of prana you are free. It is the hardest and the greatest thing to gain. You must not criticize others; you must criticize yourself. If you see a drunkard, do not criticize him; remember he is you in another shape. He who has no darkness sees no darkness in others. What you have inside you is that you see in others. This is the surest way of reform. if would-be reformers who criticize and see evil would themselves stop creating evil, the world would be better. Beat this idea into yourself.

1. Prana- in Raja Yoga

Note - Three chapters taken from Raja Yoga written by Swami Vivekananda

PranaYama is not, as many think, something about breath; breath indeed has very little to do with it, if anything. Breathing is only one of the many exercises through which we get to the real PranaYama. PranaYama means the control of "Prana. According to the philosophers of India, the whole universe is composed of two material one of which they call aksha it is the omnipresent all penetrating existence. Every thing that has form, everything that is the result of combination, is evolved out of this Akasha. It the Akasha that becomes the air, that becomes the liquids, that becomes the solids; it is the Akasha that becomes the sun, the earth, the moon, the stars, the comets; it is the Akasha that becomes the human body, the animal body, the plants, every form that we see, everything that can be sensed, everything that exists. It cannot be perceived; it is so subtle that it is beyond all ordinary perception; it can only be seen when it has become gross, has taken form. At the beginning of creation there is only this Akasha. At the end of the cycle the solids, the liquids, and the gases all melt into the Akasha again. And the next creation similarly proceeds out of this Akasha.

By what power is this aksha manufactured into this universe? by the power of prana. Just as Akasha is the infinite, omnipresent material of this universe, so is this prana the infinite, omnipresent manifesting power of this universe. At the beginning and at the end of a cycle everything becomes Akasha, and all the forces that are in the universe resolve back into the Prana; in the next cycle out of this Prana is evolved everything that we call energy everything that we call force. It is the Prana that is: manifesting as motion; it is the Prana that is manifesting' as gravitation, as magnetism.

It is the prana that is manifesting as the actions of the body, as the nerve currents as thought force. From thought down to the lowest force, every thing is but the manifestation of Prana. The sum total of all forces in the universe, mental or physical, when resolved back to their original state, is called Prana. When there was neither aught nor naught, when darkness was covering darkness, what existed then? That Akasha existed without motion; the physical motion of the Prana was stopped, but it existed all the same.

At the end of a cycle the energies now displayed in the universe quiet down and become potential. At the beginning of the next cycle they start up, strike upon the Akasha, and out of the Akasha evolve these various forms and as the, Akasha changes, this Prana changes also into all these manifestations of energy. The knowledge and control of this Prana is really what is meant by Pranayama.

This opens to us the door to almost unlimited power. Suppose, for instance, a man understood the prana perfectly, and could control it, what power on earth would not be his? He would be able to move the sun and stars out of their places, to control everything in the universe, from the atoms to' the biggest suns, because he would control the Prana. This is the end and aim of Pranayama.

When the Yogi becomes perfect; there will be nothing in nature not under his control. If he orders the gods or the souls of the departed to come, they will come at his bidding. All the forces of nature will obey him as slaves. When the ignorant see these powers of the Yogi, they call them the miracles. One peculiarity of the Hindu mind is that it always in enquires for the last possible generalization, leaving the details to be worked out afterwards.

The question is raised in the Vedas, what is that knowing which, we shall know everything? Thus, all books, and all philosophies that have been written, have been only to prove that by knowing which every thing is known. If a man wants to know this universe bit by bit, he must know every individual grain of sand, which means infinite time; he cannot know all of them. Then how can knowledge be? How is it possible for a man to be all-knowing through particulars? The yogis say that this particular manifestation there is a generalization. Behind all particular ideas stands a generalized, an abstract principle; grasp it, an you have grasped everything.

Just as this whole universe has been generalized in the Vedas into that one absolute existence and he who has grasped that existence has grasped the whole universe, so all forces have been generalized into this Prana, and he who has grasped the Prana has grasped all the forces of the universe, mental or physical. He who has controlled the Prana has controlled his own mind, and all the minds that exist. He who has controlled the Prana has controlled his body and all the bodies that exist, because the Prana is the generalized manifestation of force.

How to control the Prana is the one idea Pranayama. All the trainings and exercises in this regard are for that one end. Each man must begin where he stands, must learn how to control the things that are nearest to him. This body is very near to us, nearer than anything in the external universe and, this 'mind is the nearest of all the prana which is working this mind and body is the nearest to us of all the prana in the universe. This little wave of the Prana which represents our own energies, mental and physical, is the nearest to us of all the waves of the infinite ocean of Prana.

If we can succeed in controlling that little wave, then alone we can hope to control the whole of prana. The yogi who has done this gains perfection no longer is he under any power. He becomes almost almighty, almost all-knowing. We see sects in every country who have attempted this control of Prana. In this country there are Mind-healers, Faith-healers, Spiritualists, Christian Scientists, Hypnotists, etc., and if we examine these different bodies, we shall find at the back of each this control of the Prana, whether they know it or not. If you boil all their theories down, the residuum(balance) will be that.

It is the one and the same force they are manipulating, only unknowingly. They have stumbled on the discovery of a force and are using it unconsciously without knowing its nature, but it is the same as the Yogi uses, and which comes from Prana. ,

The Prana is the vital force in every being. Thought is the finest and highest action of prana. Thought, again, as we see, is not all. There is also what we call instinct or unconscious thought, the lowest plane of action, if a mosquito stings us, our hand will strike it automatically, instinctively. This is one expression of thought. All reflex actions of the body belong to this plane of thought. There is again the other plane of thought, the conscious. I reason, I judge, I think I see the pros and cons of certain things, yet that is not all. .We know that reason is limited.

Reason can only go to a certain extend, beyond that it cannot reach. The circle within which it runs is very very limited indeed. Yet at the same time, we find facts rush into this circle. Like the coming of comets certain things come into this circle; it is certain they come from outside the limit, although our reason cannot go beyond. The causes of the phenomena intruding themselves in this small limit are outside of this limit.

The mind can exist on a still higher plane, the super conscious. when the mind has attained to that state which is called-perfect concentration super consciousness, it goes beyond the limits of reason and comes face to face with facts which no instinct or reason can ever know. All manifestation of the subtle forces of the body, the different manifestations of Prana, if trained, give a push to the mind, help it to go up higher, and become super conscious, from where it acts.

In this universe there is one continuous substance on every plane of existence. Physically this universe is one; there is no difference between the sun and you. The scientist will tell you it is only a fiction to say the contrary. There is no real difference between the table and me; the table is one point in the mass of matter, and I another point. Each form represents, as it were, one whirlpool in the infinite ocean of matter, of which not one is constant.

Just as in a rushing stream there may be millions of whirlpools, the water in each of which is different every moment, turning round and round for a few seconds, and then passing out, replaced by a fresh quantity, so the whole universe is one constantly changing mass of matter, in which all forms of existence are so many whirlpools. A mass of matter enters into one whirlpool; Say a human body, stays there for a period becomes changed, and goes out into another, say an animal body this time, from which again after a few ears it enters into another whirlpool called a lump of mineral, it is a constant change. Not one body is constant.

There is no such thing as my body, or your body, except in words, of the one huge mass of matter, one point is called a moon, another a sun, another a man, another the earth, another a plant, another a mineral. Not one is constant, but everything is changing; matter eternally concreting and disintegrating. So it is with the mind. Matter is represented by the ether; when the action of Prana is most subtle, this very ether, in the finer state of vibration, will represent the mind, and there it will be still one unbroken mass. If you can simply get to that subtle vibration, you will see and feel that the whole universe is composed of subtle vibrations. Sometimes certain drugs have the power to take us, while as yet in the senses, to that condition.

Many of you may remember the celebrated experiment of Sir Humphrey Davy, when the laughing gas overpowered him-how, during the lecture, he remained motionless, stupefied and, after that, he said that the whole universe was made up of ideas. For the time being, as it were, the gross vibrations had ceased, and only the subtle vibrations which he called ideas, were present to him. He could only see the subtle vibrations round him; everything had become thought; the whole universe was an ocean of thought, he and everyone else had become little thought whirlpools.

Thus, even in the universe of thought we find unity, and at last, when we get to the Self, we know that the Self can only be one. Beyond the vibrations of matter is its gross and subtle aspects, beyond motion there is but one. Even in manifested motion there is only unity. These facts can no more be denied. Modern physics also has demonstrated that the sum total of the energies in the universe is the same throughout. It has also been proved that this sum total of energy exists in two forms. It becomes potential, toned down, and calmed, and next it comes out manifested as all these various forces; again it goes back to the quiet state, and again it manifests. Thus it goes on evolving and involving through eternity. The control of this Prana, as before stated, is what is called Pranayama.

The most obvious manifestation of this Prana in the human body is the motion of the lungs. If that stops, as a rule all the other manifestations of force in the body will immediately stop. But there are persons who can train themselves in such a manner that the body will on, even when this motion has stopped. There are persons who can bury themselves for days, and yet live without breathing. To reach the subtle we must take help of the grosser, and so, slowly travel towards the most subtle until we gain our point. Pranayama really means controlling this motion of the lungs, and this motion is associated with the breath. Not that breath is producing it: on the contrary it is producing breath.

This motion draws in the air by pump action. The Prana is moving the lungs, the movement of the lungs draws in the aril. So Pranayama is not breathing, but controlling that muscular power which moves the lungs. That muscular power which goes out through the nerves to the muscles and from them to the lungs, making them move in a certain manner, is the Prana, which we have to control in the practice of pranayama. When the Prana has become controlled, then we shall immediately find that all the other actions of the Prana in the body will slowly come under control. I myself have seen men who have controlled almost muscle of the body ; and why not?

If I have control over certain muscles, why not over every muscle and nerve of the body? What impossibility is there? At present the control is lost, and the motion has become automatic. We cannot move our ears at will, but we know that animals can. We have not that power because we do not exercise it. This is what is called atavism.

Again, we know that motion which has become latent can be brought back to manifestation. By hard work and practice certain motions of the body which are most dormant can be brought back under perfect control. Reasoning thus we find there is no impossibility, but, on the other hand, every probability that each part of the body can be brought under perfect control. This the yogi does through Pranayama. Perhaps some of you have read that in Pranayama, when drawing in the breath, you must fill your whole body with Prana.

In the English translations Prana is given as breath, and you are inclined to ask how that is to be done. The fault is with the translator. Every part of the body can be filled with prana, this vital force, and when you are able to do that, you can control the whole body. All the sickness and misery felt in the body will be perfectly controlled; not only so, you will be able to control another's body. Everything is infectious in this world, good or bad. If your body is in a certain state of tension, it will have a tendency to produce the same tension in others. If you are strong and and healthy, those that live near you will also have the tendency to become strong and healthy, but if you are sick and weak, those around you will have the tendency to become the same.

In the case of man trying to heal another, the first idea is simply transferring his own health to the other. This is the primitive sort of healing. Consciously or unconsciously, health can be transmitted. A very strong man, living with a weak man will make him a little stronger, whether he knows it or not. When consciously done, it becomes quicker and better in its action. Next come those cases in which a man may not be very healthy himself, yet we know that he can bring health to another. The first man, in such a case, has a little more control over the Prana and can rouse, for the time being, his Prana, as it were to a certain state of vibration, and transmit it to another person.

There have been cases where this process has been carried on at a distance, but in reality there is no distance in the sense of a break. Where is the distance that has a break? Is there any break between you and the sun? It is a continuous mass of matter, the sun being one part, and you another. Is there a break between one part of a river and another? Then why cannot any force travel, There is no reason against it. Cases of healing from a distance are perfectly true. The Prana can be transmitted to a very great distance; but to one genuine case, there are hundreds of frauds. This process of healing is not so easy as it is thought to be.

In the most ordinary cases of such healing you will find that the healers simply take advantage of the naturally healthy state of the human body. An allopath comes and treats cholera patients, and gives them his medicines. The homoeopath comes and gives his medicines, and cures perhaps more than the allopath does, because the homoeopath does not disturb his patients, but allows nature to deal with them. The Faith-healer cures more still, because he brings the strength of his mind to bear, and rouses, through faith, the dormant prana of the patient.

There is a mistake constantly made by Faith-healers: they think that faith directly heals a man. But faith alone does not cover all the ground. There are diseases where the worst symptoms are that the patient never thinks that he has that disease. That tremendous faith of the patient is itself, one symptom of the disease, and usually indicates that he will die quickly. In such cases the principle that faith cures does not apply. If it were faith alone that cured these patients also would be cured. It is by the Prana that real curing comes. The pure man, who has controlled the Prana, has the power of bringing it into a certain state of vibration, which can be conveyed to others, arousing in them a similar vibration.

You see that in everyday actions. I am talking to you. What am I trying to do? I am, so to say, bringing my mind to a certain state of vibration, and the more I succeed in bringing it to that state, the more you will be affected by what I say. All of you know that the day I am more enthusiastic, the more you enjoy the lecture; and when I am less enthusiastic, you feel lack of interest.

The gigantic will-powers of the world, the world-movers, can bring their Prana into a high state of vibration, and it is so great and powerful that it catches others in a moment and thousands are drawn towards them, and half the world thinks as they do. Great prophets of the world had the most wonderful control of the Prana, which gave them tremendous will-power; they had brought their prana to the highest state of motion, and this is what gave them power to sway the world.

All manifestations of power arise from this control. Men may not know the secret but this is the one explanation. Sometimes in your own body the supply of Prana gravitates more or less to one part; the balance is disturbed, and when the balance of prana is disturbed, what we call disease is produced.

To take away the superfluous Prana, or to supply the Prana that is wanting, will be curing the disease. That again is Pranayama—to learn when there is more or less Prana in one part of the body than there should be. The feelings will become so subtle that the mind will feel that there is less Prana in the toe or the finger than there should be, and will possess the power to supply it.

These are among the various functions of Pranayama. They have to be learned slowly and gradually, and as you see, the whole scope of Raja-Yoga is really to teach the control and direction in different planes of the Prana. When a man has concentrated his energies, he masters the Prana that is in his body. When a man is meditating, he is also concentrating the Prana.

In an ocean there are huge waves, like mountains, then smaller waves, and still smaller, down to little bubbles, but back of all these is the infinite ocean. The bubble is connected with the infinite ocean at one end, and the huge wave at the other end. So, one may be a gigantic man, and another a little bubble, but each is connected with that infinite ocean of energy, which is the common birthright of every animal that exists.

Wherever there is life, the storehouse of infinite energy is behind it. Starting as some fungus, some very minute, microscopic bubble, and all the time drawing from that infinite store house of energy, a form is changed slowly and steadily until in course of time it becomes a plant, then an animal, then man, ultimately God. This is attained through millions of aeons, but what is time? An increase of speed, an increase of struggle, is able to bridge the gulf of time. That which naturally takes a long time to accomplish can be shortened by the intensity of the action, says the Yogi. A man may go on slowly drawing in this energy from the infinite mass that exists in the universe, and, perhaps, he will require a hundred thousand years to become a Deva, and then, perhaps, five hundred thousand years to become still higher, and, perhaps, five millions of years to become perfect.

Given rapid growth, the time will be lessened. Why is it not possible, with sufficient effort, to reach this very perfection in six months or six years? There is no limit. Reason shows that. If an engine, with a certain amount of coal, runs two miles an hour, it will run the distance in less time with a greater supply of coal. Similarly, why shall not the soul, by intensifying its action, attain perfection in this very life? All beings will at last attain to that goal, we know. But who cares to wait all these millions of aeons? Why not reach it immediately, in this body even, in this human form? Why shall I not get that infinite knowledge, infinite power, now?

The ideal of the Yogi, the whole science of Yoga, is directed to the end of teaching men how, by intensifying the power of assimilation, to shorten the time for reaching perfection, instead of slowly advancing from point to point and waiting until the whole human race has become perfect. All the great prophets, saints, and seers of the world-what did they do? In one span of life they lived the whole life of humanity, traversed the whole length of time that it takes ordinary humanity to come to perfection.

In one life they perfect themselves; they have no thought

for anything else, never live a moment for any other idea, and thus the way is shortened for them. This is what is meant by concentration, intensifying the power of assimilation, thus shortening the time. Raja-Yoga is the science which teaches us how to gain the power of concentration.

What has Pranayama to do with spiritualism? Spiritualism is also a manifestation of Pranayama. If it be true that the departed spirits exist, only we cannot see them, it is quite probable that there may be hundreds and millions of them about us we can neither see, feel, nor touch. We may be continually passing and repassing through their bodies, and they do not see or feel us. It is a circle within a circle, universe within universe. We have five senses, and we represent Prana in a certain state of vibration. All beings in the same state of vibration will see one another, but if there are beings who represent Prana in a higher state of vibration, they will not be seen.

We may increase the intensity of a light until we cannot see it at all, but there may be beings with eyes so powerful that they can see such light. Again, if its vibrations are very low, we do not see a light, but there are animals that may see it, as cats and owls. Our range of vision is only one plane of the vibrations of this Prana. Take this atmosphere, for instance ; it is piled up layer on layer, but the layers nearer to the earth are denser than those above, and as you go higher the atmosphere becomes finer and finer. Or take the case of the ocean; as you go deeper and deeper the pressure of the water increases, and animals which live at the bottom of the sea can never come up, or they will be broken into pieces.

Think of the universe as an ocean of ether, consisting of layer after layer of varying degrees of vibration under the action of Prana; away from the centre the vibrations are less, nearer to it they become quicker and quicker ; one order of vibration makes one plane. Then suppose these ranges of vibrations are cut into planes, so many millions of miles one set of vibration, and then so many millions of miles another still higher set of vibration, and so on. It is, therefore, probable, that those who live on the plane of a certain state of vibration will have the power of recognizing one another, but will not recognize those above them. Yet, just as by the telescope and the

Microscope we can increase the scope of our vision, similarly we can by Yoga bring ourselves to the state of vibration of another plane, and thus enable ourselves to see what is going on there. Suppose this room is full of beings whom we do not see. They represent Prana in a certain state of vibration while we represent another. Suppose they represent a quick one, and we the opposite.

Prana is the material of which they are composed, as well as we. All are parts of the same ocean of Prana; they differ only in their rate of vibration. If I can bring myself to the quick vibration, this plane will immediately change for me: I shall not see you any more; you vanish and they appear. Some of you, perhaps, know this to be true. All this bringing of the mind into a higher state of vibration is included in one word in Yoga—Samadhi.

All these states of higher vibration, super conscious vibrations of the mind, are grouped in that one word, Samadhi, and the lower states of Samadhi give us visions of these beings. The highest grade of Samadhi is when we see the real thing, when we see the material out of which the whole of these grades of beings are composed, and that one lump of clay being known, we know all the clay in the universe.

Thus we see that Pranayama includes all that is true of spiritualism even. Similarly, you will find that wherever any sect or body of people is trying to search out anything occult and mystical, or hidden, what they are doing is really this Yoga, this attempt to control the Prana. You will find that wherever there is any extraordinary display of power, it is the manifestation of this Prana. Even the physical sciences can be included in Pranayama. What moves the steam engine?

Prana, acting through the steam. What are all these phenomena of electricity and so forth but Prana? What is physical science? The science of Pranayama, by external means. Prana, manifesting itself as mental power, can only be controlled by mental means. That part of Pranayama which attempts to control the physical manifestations of the Prana by physical means is called physical science, and that part which tries to control the manifestations of the Prana as mental force by mental means is called Raja-Yoga.

2. The Psychic Prana

According to the Yogis, there are two nerve currents in the spinal column, called Pingla and Ida, and a hollow canal called Sushumna running through the spinal cord. At the lower end of the hollow canal is what the Yogis call the "Lotus of the Kundalini". They describe it as triangular in form in which, in the symbolical language of the Yogis, there is a power called the Kundalini, coiled up.

When that Kundalini awakes, it tries to force a passage through this hollow canal, and as it rises step by step, as it were, layer after layer of the mind becomes open and all the different visions and wonderful powers come to the Yogi. When it reaches the brain, the Yogi is perfectly detached from the body and mind; the soul finds itself

Free. We know that the spinal cord is composed in a peculiar manner. If we take the figure eight horizontally there are two parts which are connected in the middle. Suppose you add eight after eight, piled one on top of the other that will represent the spinal cord. The left is the Ida, the right Pingla, and that hollow canal which runs through the centre of the spinal cord is the Sushumna.

Where the spinal cord ends in some of the lumbar vertebrae, a fine fibre moves downwards, and the canal runs up even within that fibre, only much finer. The canal is closed at the lower end, which is situated near what is called the sacral plexus, which, according to modern physiology, is triangular in form. The different plexuses that have their centres in the spinal canal can very well stand for the different "lotuses" of the Yogi.

The Yogi conceives of several centres, beginning with

the Muladharam, the basic, and ending with the Sahasraram, the thousand-petalled lotus in the brain. So, if we take these different plexuses as representing these lotuses, the idea of the Yogi can be understood very easily in the language of modem physiology. We know there are two sorts of actions in these nerve currents, one afferent, the other efferent; one sensory and the other motor; one centripetal, and the other centrifugal. One carries the sensations to the brain, and the other from the brain to the outer body. These vibrations are all connected with the brain in the long run.

Several other facts we have to remember, in order to clear the way for the explanation which is to come. This spinal cord, at the brain, ends in a sort of bulb, in the medulla, which is not attached to the brain, but floats in a fluid in the brain, so that if there be a blow on the head the force of that blow will be dissipated in the fluid, and will not hurt the bulb. This is an important fact to remember. Secondly, we have also to know that, of all the centres, we have particularly to remember three, the Muladharam (the basic), the Sahasraram (the thousand-petalled lotus of the brain) and the Manipurakam (the lotus of the navel).

Next we shall take one fact from physics. We all hear of electricity and various other forces connected with if. What electricity is no one knows, but so far as it is known, it is a sort of motion. There are various other motions in the universe; what is the difference between them and electricity? Suppose this table move—that the molecules which compose this table are moving in different directions; if they are all made to move in the same direction, it will be through electricity. Electric motion makes the molecules of a body move in the same direction.

If all the air molecules in a room 'are made to move in the same direction, it will make a gigantic battery of electricity of the room. Another point from physiology we must remember, that the centre which regulates the respiratory system, the breathing system, has a sort of controlling action over the system of nerve currents.

Now we shall see why breathing is practiced. In the first place, from rhythmical breathing comes a tendency of all the molecules in the body to move in the same direction. When mind changes into will, the nerve currents change into a motion similar to electricity, because the Nerves have been proved to show polarity under the action of electric currents. This shows that when the will is transformed into the nerve currents, it is changed into something like electricity.

When all the motions of the body have become perfectly rhythmical, the body has, as it were, become a gigantic battery of will. This tremendous will is exactly what the Yogi wants. This is, therefore, a physiological explanation of the breathing exercise. It tends to bring a rhythmic action in the body, and helps us, through the respiratory centre, to control the other centres. The aim of Pranayama here is to rouse the Coiled-up power in the Muladharam, called the Kundalini.

Everything that we see, or imagine, or dream, we have to perceive in space. This is the ordinary space, called the Mahakasha, or elemental space. When a Yogi reads the thoughts of other men, or perceives super-sensuous objects, he sees them in another sort of space called the Chittakasha, the mental space. When perception has become objectless, and the soul shines in its own nature, it is called the Chidakasha, or knowledge space.

When the Kundalini is aroused, and enters the canal of the Sushumna, all the perceptions are in the mental space. When it has reached that end of the canal which opens out into the brain, the objectless perception is in the knowledge space. Taking the analogy of electricity, we find that man can send a current only along a wire, but nature requires no wires to send her tremendous currents. (Note: The reader should remember that this was spoken before the discovery" of wireless telegraphy)

This proves that the wire is not really necessary, but only our inability to dispense with it compels us to us. Similarly, all the sensations and motions of the are being sent into the brain, and sent out of it, through these wires of nerve fibres. The columns of sensory and motor fibres in the spinal cord are the Ida and Pingla of the Yogis. They are the main channels through which the afferent and efferent currents travel. But why should not the mind send news without any wire, or react without any wire? We see this is done in nature. The Yogi says, if you can do that, you have got rid of the bondage of matter. How to do it?

If you can make the current pass through the Sushumna, the canal in the middle of the spinal column, you have solved the problem. The mind has made this network of the nervous system, and has to break it, so that no wires will be required to work through. Then alone will all knowledge come to us—no more bondage of body; that is why it is so important that we should get control of that Sushumna. If we can send the mental current through the hollow canal without nerve fibres to act as wires, the Yogi says, the problem is solved, and he also says it can be done.

This Sushumna is in ordinary persons closed up at the lower extremity; no action comes through it. The Yogi proposes a practice by which it can be opened, and the nerve currents made to travel through. When a sensation is carried to a centre, the centre reacts. This reaction in the case of automatic centres, is followed by motion the case of conscious centres it is followed first by perception, and secondly by motion. All perception is the reaction to action from outside. How, then, do perceptions in dreams arise? There is then no action from outside. The sensory motions, therefore, are' coiled up some where.

For instance, I see a city; the perception of that city is from the reaction to the sensations brought from outside objects comprising that city. That is to say a certain motion in the brain molecules has been set up by the motion in the in carrying nerves, which again are set in motion by external objects in the city. Now, even after a long time I can remember the city. This memory is exactly the same phenomenon, only it is in a milder form. But whence is the action that sets up even the milder form of similar vibrations in the brain? Not certainly from the primary sensations. Therefore it must be that the sensations are coiled up somewhere, and they, by their acting, bring out the mild reaction which we call dream perception.

Now the centre where all these residual sensations are, as it were, stored up, is called the Muladharam, the root receptacle, and the coiled-up energy of action is Kundalini, "the coiled up". It is very probable that the residual motor energy is also stored up in the same centre, as, after deep study or meditation on external objects, the part of the body where the Muladharam centre is situated probably the sacral plexus gets heated. Now, if this coiled-up energy be roused and made active, and then consciously made to travel up the Sushumna canal, as it acts upon centre after centre, a tremendous reaction will set in.

When a minute portion of energy travels along a nerve fibre and causes reaction from centres, the perception is either dream or imagination. But when by the power of long internal meditation the vast mass of energy stored up travels along the Sushumna, and strikes the centres, the reaction is tremendous, immensely superior to the reaction of dream or imagination, immensely more intense than the reaction of sense-perception. It is super-sensuous perception. And when it reaches the metropolis of all sensations, the brain, the whole brain, as it were, reacts, and the result is the full blaze of illumination, the perception of the Self.

As this Kundalini force travels from centre to centre, layer after layer of the mind, as it were, opens up, and this universe is perceived by the Yogi in its fine, or causal form. Then alone the causes of this universe, both as sensation and reaction, are known as they are, and hence comes all knowledge. The causes being known, the knowledge of the effects is sure to follow.

Thus the rousing of the Kundalini is the one and only way to attaining Divine Wisdom, super conscious perception, realisation of the spirit. The rousing may come in various ways, through love for God, through the mercy of perfected sages, or through the power of the analytic will of the philosopher. Wherever there was any, manifestation of what is ordinarily called supernatural power or wisdom, there a little current of Kundalini must have found its way into the Sushumna. Only, in the vast majority of such cases, people had ignorantly stumbled on some practice which set free a minute portion of the coiled-up Kundalini.

All worship, consciously or unconsciously, leads to this end. The man who thinks that he is receiving response to his prayers does not know that the fulfillment comes from his own nature, that he has succeeded by the mental attitude of prayer in waking up a bit of this infinite power which is coiled up within himself. What, thus, men ignorantly worship under various names, through fear and tribulation, the Yogi declares to the world to be the real power coiled up in every being, the mother of eternal happiness, if we but know how to approach her. And Raja-Yoga is the science of religion, the rationale of all worship, all prayers, forms, ceremonies and miracles.

3. The Control Of Psychic Prana

We have now to deal with the exercises in Pranayama. We have seen that the first step, according to the Yogis, is to control the motion of the lungs. What we want to do is to feel the finer motions that are going on in the body. Our minds have become externalized, and have lost Sight of the fine motions inside. If we can begin to feel them, we can begin to control them. These nerve currents go on all over the body, bringing life and vitality to every muscle, but we do not feel them. The Yogi says we can learn to do so. How? By taking up and

Controlling the motion of the lungs; when we have done that for a sufficient length of time, we shall be able to control the finer motions.

We now come to the exercises in Pranayama. Sit up right; the body must be kept straight. The spinal cord, although not attached to the vertebral column, is yet inside of it. If you sit crookedly you disturb this spinal cord, so let it be free. Any time that you sit crookedly and try to meditate you do yourself an injury. The three parts of the body, the chest, the neck, and the head, must be always held straight in one line. You will find that by a little practice this will come to you as easy as breathing.

The second thing is to get control of the nerves. We have said that the nerve centre that controls the respiratory organs has a sort of controlling effect on the other nerves, and rhythmical breathing is, therefore, necessary. The breathing that we generally use should not be called breathing at all. It is very irregular. Then there are some natural differences of breathing between men and women.

The first lesson is just to breathe in a measured way, in and out. That will harmonize the system. When you have practiced this for some time, you will do well to join it the repetition of some word as "Om," or any other sacred word. In India we use certain symbolical words instead of counting one, two, three, four. That is why I advise you to join the mental repetition of the "Om," or some other sacred word to the Pranayama.

Let the word flow in and out with the breath, rhythmically, harmoniously, and you will find the whole body is becoming rhythmical. Then you will learn what rest is. Compared with it, sleep is not rest. Once this rest comes the most tired nerves will be calmed down, and you will find that you have never before really rested. The first effect of this practice is perceived in the change of expression of one's face; harsh lines disappear, with calm thought calmness comes over the face. Next comes the beautiful voice. I never saw a Yogi with a croaking voice. These signs come after a few months practice.

After practicing the above mentioned breathing for a few days, you should take up a higher one. Slowly fill the lungs with breath through the Ida, the left nostril, and at the same time concentrate the mind on the nerve current. You are, as it were, sending the nerve current down the spinal column, and striking violently on the last plexus, the basic lotus which is triangular in form, the seat of the Kundalini. Then hold the current there for some time.

Imagine that you are slowly drawing that nerve current with the breath through the other side, the Pingla, then slowly throw it out through the right nostril. This you will find a little difficult to practice. The easiest way is to stop the right nostril with the thumb, and then slowly draw in the breath through the left; then close both nostrils with thumb and forefinger, and imagine that you are sending that current down, and striking the base of the Sushumna ; then take the thumb off, and let the breath out through the right nostril. Next inhale slowly through nostril, keeping the other closed by the forefinger, then close both, as before.

The way the Hindus practice this would be very difficult for this country, because they do it from their childhood, and their lungs are prepared for it. Here it is well to begin with four seconds, and slowly increase. Draw in four seconds, hold in sixteen seconds, then throw out in eight seconds. This makes one Pranayama. At the same time think of the basic loutus, triangular in form; concentrate the mind on that centre. The imagination can help you a great deal. The next breathing is slowly drawing the breath in, and then immediately throwing it out slowly, and then stopping the breath out, using the same numbers. The only difference is that in the first case the breath was held in, and in the second, held out. This last is the easier one.

The breathing in which you hold the breath in the lungs must not be practiced too much. Do it only four times in the morning, and four times in the evening. Then you can slowly increase the time and number. You will find that you have the power to do so, and that you take pleasure in it. So very carefully and cautiously increase as you feel that you have the power, to six instead of four. It may injure you if you practice it irregularly.

Of the three processes for the purification of the nerves, described above, the first and the last are neither difficult nor dangerous. The more you practice the first one the calmer you will be. Just think of "Om," and you can practice even while you are sitting at your work. You will be all the better for it. Some day, if you practice hard, the Kundalini will be aroused. For those who practice once or twice a day, just a little calmness of the body and mind will come, and beautiful voice; only for those who can go on further with it will Kundalini be aroused, and the whole of nature will begin to change, and the book of Knowledge will open. No more will you need to go to books for knowledge; your own mind will have become your book, containing infinite knowledge.

I have already spoken of the Ida and Pingla currents, flowing through either side of the spinal column, and also of the Sushumna, the passage through the centre of the spinal cord. These three are present in every animal; whatever being has a spinal column has these three lines of action. But the Yogis claim that in an ordinary man the Sushumna is closed; its action is not evident while that of the other two is carrying power to different parts of the body.

The Yogi alone has the Sushumna open. When this Sushumna current opens, and begins to rise, we get beyond the sense, our minds become super sensuous, super conscious—we get beyond even the intellect, where reasoning cannot reach. To open that Sushumna is the prime object of the Yogi. According to him, along this Sushumna are ranged these centres, or, in more figurative language, these lotuses, as they are called. The lowest one is at the lower end of the spinal cord, and is called Muladharam, the next higher is called Swadhistanam, the third Manipurakam, the fourth Anahatam, the fifth Vishudhi, the sixth Aagnya and the last, which is in the brain, is -the Sahasraram, or "the thousand-petalled".

Of these we have to take cognition just now of two centres only, the lowest, the Muladharam, and the highest, the Sahasraram. All energy has to be taken up from its seat in the Muladharam and brought to the Sahasraram. The Yogis claim that of all the energies that are in the human body the highest is what they call "Ojas". Now this Ojas is stored up in the brain, and the more Ojas is in a man's head, the more powerful he is, the more intellectual, the more spiritually strong.

One man may speak beautiful language and beautiful thoughts, but they do not impress people; another man speaks neither beautiful language nor beautiful thoughts, yet his words charm. Every movement of his is powerful. That is the power of Ojas. Now in every man there is more or less of this Ojas Stored up. All the forces that are working in the body in their highest become Ojas. You must remember that, it is only a question of transformation. The same force which is working outside as electricity or magnetism will become changed into inner force; the same forces that are working as muscular energy will be changed into Ojas.

The Yogis say that that part of the human energy which is expressed as sex energy, in sexual thought, when checked and controlled, easily becomes changed into Ojas, and as the Muladharam guides these, the Yogi pays particular attention to that centre. He tries to take up all his sexual energy and convert it into Ojas. It is only the chaste man or woman who can make the Ojas rise and store it in the brain; that is why chastity has always been considered the highest virtue.

A man feels that if he is unchaste, spirituality goes away; he loses mental vigor and moral stamina. That is why in all the religious orders in the world which have produced spiritual giants you will always find absolute chastity insisted upon. That is why the monks came into existence, giving up marriage. There must be perfect chastity in thought, word, and deed; without it the practice of Raja-Yoga is dangerous, and may lead to insanity. If people practice Raja-Yoga and at the same time lead an impure life, how can they expect to become Yogis?"

Reiki Manuals

Level One & Two

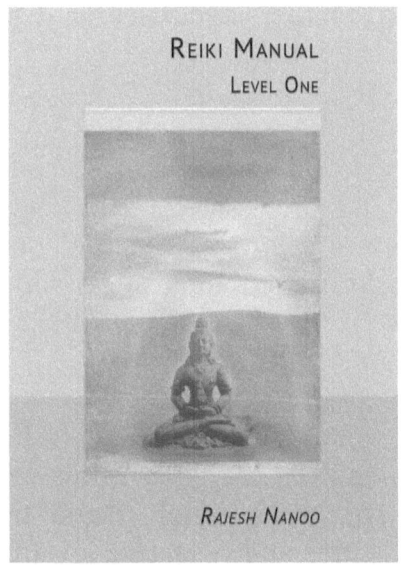
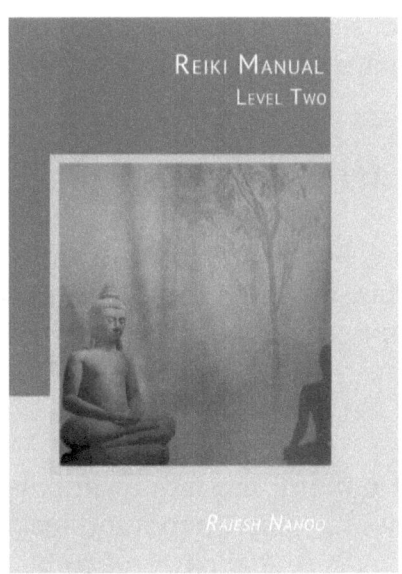

Paperbacks and EBooks are available in Createspace, Amazon, Lulu, Smashwords etc. Contact author website for more details.

www.rajeshnanoo.com

Other Books

1. The Cave Of Wisdom

The Book contains the gist of mystical teachings from Upanishads, Zen, Sufism, Kabbala, Buddhism and Taoism. Along with this, it covers the very essence of Semitic philosophy that is spread through Christianity, Islam and Judaism.

The book has many verses and stories of Upanishad exclusively translated by the author. The principal ideologies said by Upanishad Saints are shared in the book.

2. Wine Of Words

This book contains 100 short verses of progressive ideology. These thoughts aroused from Zen, Sufi, and Kabbalistic wisdom baptized in Vedantic doctrines.

3. Be......

31 mindful matters to middle path. All the good things are possible only when mind feels inspired. The whole idea of the book is to make people to be reflective and receptive towards every situations of life.

4. Reiki Sutras

Reiki the vibrational energy medicine when emitted through hands of Healer whose mind meditating on subtle love realms have the potential to relax, rejuvenate and renovate any human body and subtle bodies. The book explores the pillars and healing methodology of Reiki, which was built from the foundation laid by Saints in Indian Tantra and Lamas from Buddhism.